30 Day Shred Diet Concept

Introductory Fast Weight Loss Book toward Permanent Health & Wellness

By Cathy Wilson
Copyright © 2014

Income Disclaimer

This book contains business strategies, marketing methods and other business advice that, regardless of my own results and experience, may not produce the same results (or any results) for you. I make absolutely no guarantee, expressed or implied, that by following the advice below you will make any money or improve current profits, as there are several factors and variables that come into play regarding any given business.

Primarily, results will depend on the nature of the product or business model, the conditions of the marketplace, the experience of the individual, and situations and elements that are beyond your control.

As with any business endeavor, you assume all risk related to investment and money based on your own discretion and at your own potential expense.

Liability Disclaimer

By reading this book, you assume all risks associated with using the advice given below, with a full understanding that you, solely, are responsible for anything that may occur as a result of putting this information into action in any way, and regardless of your interpretation of the advice.

You further agree that our company cannot be held responsible in any way for the success or failure of your business as a result of the information presented in this book. It is your responsibility to conduct your own due diligence regarding the safe and successful operation of your business if you intend to apply any of our information in any way to your business operations.

Terms of Use

You are given a non-transferable, "personal use" license to this book. You cannot distribute it or share it with other individuals.

Also, there are no resale rights or private label rights granted when purchasing this book. In other words, it's for your own personal use only.

30 Day Shred Diet Concept

Introductory Fast Weight Loss Book toward Permanent Health & Wellness

By Cathy Wilson

Table of Contents

Introduction

I'm convinced as humans, we are intrinsically programmed to NEVER, ever in a zillion million years be
totally and unwaveringly happy with our body. It doesn't
matter if you are a 6 foot pencil thin 110 pound model, an
Angelina Jolie lookalike or the fittest 40 year-old on the
planet. We always seem to want what we don't have, regardless of what it is and never stopping to smell the
roses and consider what we do have.

Sound eerily familiar?
Hence our fad diet world is a multi-trillion dollar industry
thriving and so very alive. Consider into the equation, we
couldn't be further away from the lifestyle our "cavemen"
ancestors lived through. Where physical activity, the fittest of the fit was how it was. Every single thing they had
and did was centered around getting physical. Funny
how the tune, "Let's get physical...physical...I wanna get
physical..." just popped into my head.

When hungry, rustic, manly cave- men hopped on their
horses or by foot and went tracking wild game. If they
were lucky, after hours of intense cardiovascular and
strength training activities, squatting, sprinting, jogging,
dodging, squeezing and jumping, they were about to take
down an elephant of gazelle, again, with physical effort,
after which, they had to drag the unlucky, dead weight of
meat back to camp 4 or 5 miles away. It was, then
cleaned and cooked and before that happened, out again
the men went to gather the firewood, grasses and anything else required to burn a beautiful fire in which to
cook the prize. Of course, there were also side dishes
that needed to first be found in the forest, then cleaned

and prepared. All required oodles of physical and strenu-
ously tiring exertion.

NEWSFLASH!

This is how the human body is meant to function, with
plenty of physically challenging exercise EVERY DAY. A
heck of a lot more than the measly 30-60 minute we tell
ourselves today is adequate. Adequate for what? To
keep from turning into a bump on the log?
Add to this the healthy CLEAN, non-toxic, pesticide-free,
good fats, no simple high sugar carb diet with plenty of
essential vitamins, minerals and fiber. And you've got
one healthy dude or dudette!

Obviously, you'd look a little silly putting on your loin
cloth, hopping on your horse and bolting down the city
street in search of what? Birds? Wild Dogs? Maybe the
odd stray fox? Yes, you'd end up in the slammer for trying to do the "right" thing for your mind and body.
Is there a perfect solution? Nope. Sorry to say, the times
have changed and there's no use crying over spilt milk.

FACT!
We are a lazy ass society looking to cut corners in everything we do. We really don't care about Mother Nature
and the world we live in. All we want is MORE, MORE
and then a little MORE.

Seeing is believing. Look around you and just try and ar-
gue with me. Of course I'm talking in general terms
because there are always exceptions to the rules. My
many years on this planet has taught me that.

For over TWENTY years I have studied, eaten and
breathed health and wellness. I've learned by reading,
writing, listening and most importantly doing. And with

every single diet concept I have studied and tested, there's always something positive to take from it. At least one piece of useful information you can take and store in your noggin to use in your never-ending quest to drop that last 10 or 20 pounds from your fed-up frame.

This introductory book is going to look specifically into the 30 Shred Diet and discuss with you the pros and cons and whether or not this a weight loss concept that needs my magic wand to work, which of course, is in the shop right now – UGH! We are focusing on the "physical" side of the equation of good health for life. That's the cardio-vascular, muscle building, toning, strengthening and stretching side.

This 30 Day Shred Diet concept is claimed to be devised by Jillian Michaels, who make her way to fame as the nu-tritionist on the reality show "The Biggest Loser." (I'm pretty sure anyway!) Another name you might be familiar with that is connected with this "concept" is Alexandria Foster. This exercise program is separate from the eating end of the equation. A 6 week diet program labelled "The Shred Diet," by Ian Smith. With the idea of confusing your tummy with food diversity and constant, controlled eating to kick start the metabolism and encourage continuous fat burning at the highest level.

We'll touch a little on that diet plan, but our focus is on the exercise portion of the "30 Day Shred Diet."
Time for you to open your mind. Use your assumed logic and take from this informational introduction book to help get that last 10-20 pounds off your crying body and make it smile for real. Understanding the positive health chang-es you make need to be for life. Temporary doesn't' work with weight loss. Your head needs to be on straight.

DECIDE you are going to do whatever it takes to lose
that pesky last few pounds and continue to do whatever it
takes FOREVER to keep it off.
Let's get started if you're ready?

Key Factors in Losing Ten to Twenty Pounds

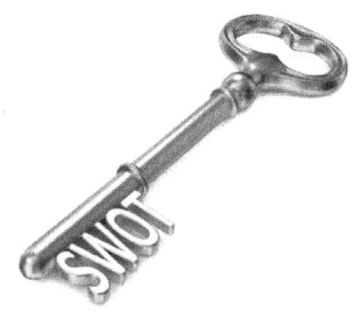

Losing weight doesn't have to be tough to figure out. But it will be hard to implement simply because we are creatures of habit and just hate to make changes. Even if the changes are going to help boost self-esteem, increase energy, strength and tone our body, deter illness and disease, diminish annoying aches and pains and help us flip our life switch to positive if it requires changes in our troubling and unhealthy lifestyle habits. We revert to saying "talk to the hand," even when we half convince ourselves to start making better nutrition choices and hit the gym at least on occasion. More often than not, we allow excuses to get in the way. We veer of our new roughly cut path and crash straight through the door of the house that contains all our old nasty and unproductively debilitating habits. The sad part is we are often happy to arrive back in our comfort zone.

Make the choice to throw all your built-in self-sabotaging excuses out the window for good and start looking for the life changes that might work with you in blasting fat and getting skinny happy.

The "National Weight Control Registry" has conducted research studies to determine just what characteristics are constant in the lives of people that have lost those last few pounds you are looking to banish. They have the "goods" on weight loss you're looking for and I'm going to use this information to help educate you on what needs to change and how you can do it in order to lower your scale number and keep it there. This may or may not involve concepts from the "30 Day Shred Diet." We'll look into that part a little later.

CRITICAL KEYS IF YOU'RE SERIOUS ABOUT FLUBBY FAT LOSS FOR GOOD!

Commit Your Head

Don't fake it here or I can tell you right now you might as well hop on the bandwagon of "yo-yo" dieting right now. You are in charge of you and YOU make your own choices in life. Turn left, right or drive straight through the barricade? Get caught and you can't have your friend head down to the station instead of you.

The point is, only serious people succeed in permanent weight loss, a commitment of making new, healthier habits for LIFE. Not a few days, months or years. This is all about forever. Till death do you part. Understanding it's a whole whack of hard work, perseverance and commitment to change up front. Then, you're rewarded because it does get easier and eventually you'll naturally be looking for ways to get healthier.

How do I know this?

Simply, because I live it and take a look at me. Seeing is believing.

Cathy Facts:

-Gave birth to SIX children

-5'7", 110 lbs
-Extremely fit, lean and muscular with low body fat (6 pack to prove it!)
-eat healthy and exercise 5-6 days a week for an hour
The point is, if you train your mind and body to be healthy, the maintaining part of the equation is a piece of cake. Understand, this will take time, mistakes and successes. Keep one foot in front of the other, never quitting and you WILL reach your goals if that's what you choose. If you want it, you can have it. Just make sure you're the committing type or just don't bother.

Open Your Mind to Find Balance in Eating
There are so many dieting experts out there telling you all sorts of supposed "scientifically proven" strategies of eating to lose weight. Read, listen and learn to all of them, but keep in mind it's all about balance. Nothing should be completely discluded from your eating plan. Simply, because you need to work with your body over time and figure out what food combinations work best for you.

Perhaps, you seem to metabolize protein more efficiently and effectively than good carbohydrates, which may bung you up a little. Take this information and use it to your advantage. You know you need complex carbs to maintain good health. You just might be on the lower end of the scale of 4-8 servings per day for optimal health. Are you following what I'm saying?

Most of the people from this fat loss registry study, which is ample proof in my books. Eat a fairly low calorie diet consisting of up to 1400 calories, depending on their activity level, body makeup and weight loss goals. They also surprisingly get about half of their calories from complex carbs, like veggies, fruits and healthy whole grain products, beans and lentils. Next, comes almost 20% from muscle building, cell building and maintenance, energy rich protein. Making up the rear is almost 25% of daily calories coming from healthy fats. This means un-saturated fats, including avocado, nuts, vegetable oils and an exception to the rule here, coconut products. The basics, anyway.

Often, the issue is people eat too much of the wrong foods and not enough of the right. Your body is forgiving and if you happen to indulge a little too much with "healthy" foods, it's not going to be as devastating as too many fast-food drive-thru's, theater popcorn, soda, chips and Twinkies!

The bottom line is, researchers have re-discovered a basic low-fat and high "healthy' carbohydrate diet fits the bill for long-term weight loss.

You've Gotta Get Sweaty and Eventually LOVE It!
Just take your thoughts back to the introduction where we talked about how it used to be a way, way back in time. Exercising regularly is a necessary and ingrained part of your physiological makeup. It's always been there and always will be. Your health problems have manifest-ed because you've either ignored this fact or not been consistent with exercising. Here and there just doesn't cut it. Going nuts around April/May to get ready for swim-suit season is a joke. You know and I know come winter time you'll act like a lazy bear and pack on the pounds for hibernation.

WAKEUP CALL...You Are NOT A Bear. So STOP Acting Like One!!!
Back to the Weight Loss Registry data. These people re-ported up to an hour and a half a day. My first thoughts? TOO MUCH!

Don't fret though, because it all depends upon what type of exercise you are doing and at what exertion rate, if you are intensely training, like in a boot camp session, where you're interval training with weights and cardio and maximizing your efforts. Then less time is required to get more results, if, however, you are coasting along on your bike at a moderate pace for 90 minutes hardly breaking a sweat. Then yes, you will need a longer exercise time to burn the number of calories you are aiming for each day that will aid you in dropping your fat rolls. Again, it's your choice.

Myself, I prefer hard and short, a hard interval training regimen often rotated between the spin-bike, elliptical trainer and running, with heavy weights, forced reps to maximize my strength training. A half hour to 45 minutes cardio and 15 minutes weights is all she wrote for me. But, I make sure I'm challenged and push myself hard each and every workout.

Works for me!
Always run your exercise idea through your doctor before starting just to be safe. And make sure you start off slow in whatever you do. Building yourself up with time to get happy and get results with your diverse and effective exercise regimen.
Again, we'll look into the 30 Day Shred Diet a little later.

Fuel Your Body Consistently – Starting With Breakfast
I'm sure you've heard that breakfast is the most important meal of the day. IT IS! When you wake your body is running on empty and if you want to set your physical and mental up for success you need to replenish your supplies. Can't drive your car on empty, so why in heck's name would you try it with your body? This is a learned thing and if you have learned not to eat in the morning

you need to unlearn it. And learn that you WILL be eating breakfast from this day on forever if you're serious about losing fat, keeping it off and getting healthy.

Research also shows more benefits of filling your tummy with healthy foods pronto in the morning are:
-Better energy levels
-Clearer and more focused/productive thinking
-Improved mood
-Lower cholesterol levels
-Helps maximize the metabolic rate
-Sets you up to eat less during the day
-Less risk of "pig-out" sessions because blood sugars are level

Getting a good breakfast with lean protein to nip your hungry feeling in the bud and the energy your body needs for lean muscle building and cell maintenance and repair. Eggs are a great choice or perhaps ham. Most milk products are good protein sources too, just careful of the fat content. Also, include complex carbohydrates to give you the fiber you need to feel full and help flush harmful toxins from your system, along with giving you long term energy. Whole grain breads and cereals are great. As opposed to simple carbs, white breads, cakes and pastries. Which provide little to no nutritional value and a short burst of energy that sends you plummeting back down to the bottom of the energy barrel fast and furiously. Meaning grabbing a donut or packaged pastry on your way to work is futile. Take two minutes to toast some whole grain toast, add a smear of peanut butter and grab a banana. You can get your non-fat latte on the way to work and you're all set!

It's also critical to teach your body to trust that you are going to feed it regularly. How do you do this?

By making sure you eat regularly, every 3-4 hours in small amounts. Balanced mini-meals are best because they give your internal systems a constant supply of energy to function optimally. Eating healthy and regular will also help stabilize blood sugars, a deterrent for developing diabetes, which is a serious blood sugar disorder.

Learn to Make Healthier Food Choices in the Right Amounts
If you really want to lose fat and keep it off. Something has to give. You're insane if you think you can keep on doing the same thing and get different results. So, if you're used to eating a candy bar and soda for your morning snack and expect to lose weight, then you're wise to ditch both and have a handful of nuts, banana and a yogurt, with crisp and refreshing water to drink. More food with less calories, providing the protein, good carbs, fats, vitamins and minerals your body needs to burn fat and reek energy!

You need to relearn how to eat. Ditching the fast-foods; high fats, bad fats, high simple surgery carbs, low vitamin and mineral count foods. And opt for filling your tummy up with adequate amounts of lean meat protein, energy extending complex good carbs, good unsaturated fats, vitamins, minerals and adequate hydration (water), to maximize the performance of your body mentally, physically and spiritually.

Removing that crap foods from your diet will remove the interference in your good health. Your energy levels will remain constant and pure. Laziness and grogginess will be a thing of the past. Foggy thinking, annoying aches and pains, along with bouts of depression and extreme anxiety will dissipate.
TRUTH??

Every single healthier eating choice you learn and practice into habit, will help you look, feel, act and BE a better person.

How do you do this?

One step at a time. Start slow and keep on making the changes, repeating them until they are concrete and co-operating with your new healthier way of thinking, just to give you an idea. Repeating one new action regularly for at least THREE months straight will get you to the edge of the turning point where you can call it a habit. You'll know when you hit this point because you won't have to "think" about choosing whole grain pasta with tomato sauce and grilled chicken instead of white cheesy pasta with deep fried crispy chicken. Grabbing a bowl of oatmeal in the morning with a handful of nuts and banana, instead of a vending machine muffin and soda will be a no-brainer. I hope this is making sense to you.

One change at a time and a commitment to make positive eating changes and allow for the odd slip up is how it's gotta be. You're creating your new blueprint for life here. Time and patience are a MUST, a give and take relationship full of comprises that work for you personally. For example, Maybe, you just can't go without you theater popcorn when you hit the movie theater about every two weeks? Ok. Have your popcorn, but try and make a few modifications. A few things to consider...

*Order extra small and eat it slowly
*Share it with a friend
*Make sure you eat a healthy snack before the movies so you're less hungry
*Try switching to another "more healthy" treat, like licorice or a small bag of chips
*Get an extra hour of cardiovascular exercise in before or after the movies for damage control

As you can see, there are lots of different routes for you to have your treat and still stay on track with your goals. The mental and just "thinking" you are progressing is so very important to long-term success.

Keep your mind open and always be looking for eating strategies you can implement that will help you make better eating choices. "Healthier" doesn't happen overnight. It needs continuous maintenance and betterment if you truly want it to last a lifetime. You game to commit to that?

My Thoughts…

It's no secret that you control you. If you truly want to make the changes necessary to vamoose that last pesky 20-30 pounds, you will! Open your mind and look for what works with your preferences and tolerances. Accept getting healthy and losing weight takes time, perseverance and the ability to muck up and get yourself back on track. Chin up. You've already taken the first step toward showing a desire to make positive change. Onward you go!

Physiological – How Your Body Burns Calories

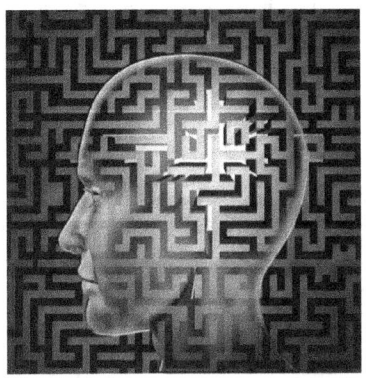

It's a no-brainer that if you want to lose weight, to drop that bothersome last 10-20 pounds, that's been weighing you down for what seems like forever. You've got to understand at least the basics of how your body works. How it burns calories and zaps fat.

Your metabolism is the star of the show here.
The metabolism is directly linked to your weight by having a naturally "slower" or "faster" metabolism isn't the deciding factor in whether or not you have the "ability" to lose weight. It will just slightly affect the length of time it will take for you to accomplish your weight loss goals. Just make the choice to deal with it. No excuses allowed here.

According to *The Mayo Clinic*, it's your exercise and eating habits that decide your weight and whether or not you're going to reach your weight loss goal and keep that weight off for good.

Looking a touch further into the basics of all this…

WHAT IS METABOLISM?
It's the process in which your body converts the fuel you provide, food, into usable energy for your daily energy needs. This includes your physical exercise, walking, smiling, running, jumping. Along with the internal needs like organ function, breathing, and other processes that keep your body ticking.

Throughout this biological process of metabolism, the calories in the food and drink you feed your body releases energy for your body to use, even when sleeping your body is still burning energy for automated processes like cell restoration and blood circulation.
Your Basal Metabolic Rate is the number of calories your body uses to maintain its lowest level of energy needs. This isn't factoring in any exercise you might do. This number reflects the number of calories you'd need if you just slept all day.

Your BMR is reflective of:
-Age
-Sex
-Genetic Makeup
-Height, Weight and Body Composition
This basic rate of burning energy makes up approximately seventy-five percent of your total caloric or energy needs.

Two other key factors in the rate in which you burn calories are:
-Thermogenesis or the Processing of Food – digestion, absorption, processing and transport of energy to your internal systems.
-Exercise – walking, biking, hiking, weight training etc.

Your metabolism is a natural process and you pretty much have no choice other than to work with the metabolism you have. There are strategies you can implement that will help encourage a higher rate of energy burn.

Tips to Gently Nudge Your Metabolism Higher
Eat Breakfast
Increase Lean Protein
Choose Low Glycemic Foods
Easy On the Carbs
Focus On Antioxidant Rich Green Tea
Eat Mini-Meals
Exercise Regularly
Focus On Building Lean Muscle
LISTEN To Your Body and Eat Sensibly When You're Hungry

But, the bottom line is you need to adjust your nutrition intake and increase your physical exercise to knock off those extra spare tires. It takes determination, perseverance and a commitment to do whatever it takes to make it happen. All for life!

Please note there are medical conditions that can interfere with the rate in which the body burns calories. These are rare and of course, make it that much more difficult to lose weight naturally. Hypothyroidism and Cushing's syndrome are examples. If you suspect you have a serious metabolic condition, go get the official diagnosis. There are no excuses for not being able to lose those extra pounds otherwise. And even if you do have a very rare metabolic condition, it's just going to be a little harder for you, but it still can be done if that's what you CHOOSE to do.

Exercising and eating better are two controllable and extremely necessary factors in teaching your body to burn rather than store extra calories and help to optimize your weight loss efforts, leaving you slim, sexy, more energetic and physiologically sound than if you got lazy and didn't bother trying to lose the weight. Again, it's all a personal choice.

My Thoughts…

Understanding the importance of your metabolism and how your body burns calories and fat, is critical in making the right choices for you to drop weight. The bottom line is, calorie expenditure has to be greater than calorie intake at the end of the day. If you understand that you are on your way to a sexier, slimmer, more energized and bodaciously beautiful you.

Bare Bones – Why You Need Exercise

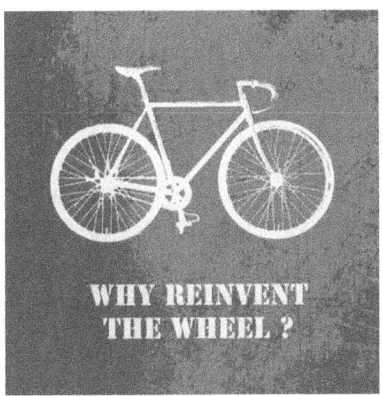

WHY REINVENT
THE WHEEL ?

Boy, do we seem to look for excuses here. Trying to find reasons to justify not exercising instead of just doing it and not needing the nuts and bolts of why your body physiologically needs to be constantly building energy and challenging the level in which you can get oxygen to your vital organs.

Exercise benefits you mentally and physically, and is the one thing in life you have control over. Something that can help you live a happier, healthier and more productively fantabulous life as a whole. If you need the science of it, exercise helps to improve your mood by releasing those natural happy drugs, endorphins, to make you feel high on life. It will make you look better and routine muscle building and cardiovascular training also helps deter the natural breakdown of the body, disease and any other interference factors that just might cut your life short.

Exercise Benefits…

MOOD – Naturally encourages hormone release that makes your mind and body feel happy, happy, happy!

LONGER Life – Regular exercise helps to maintain optimal function of your body, making it more resilient and likely to last longer than the energizer bunny.

PROTECTS – Keeping your blood pumping protects from serious disease and illness including heart disease, stroke and diabetes to start.

HELPS DETER BONE LOSS – With the inevitable aging process comes the natural breakdown of bone. Bone loss in serious amounts is labelled osteoporosis and regular strength training and cardiovascular activity help protect from this disease.

HELPS STABALIZE AND KEEP MOBILE – Keeping your limbs nimble, agile and limber is only going to help you stay steady on your feet and move flexible and bendable in general. Reaching up for the jars on the top shelf of the cupboard isn't going to cause you any pain if you're taking care of your body.

HELPS CONTROL WEIGHT PLUS – Routine physical activity encourages weight loss, helps keep it off and deters those extra pounds from creeping back on. But only if you commit to it for life!

BETTERS SLEEP – It's not a deep, dark secret that researchers have documented exercise on a regular basis promotes a quality nights rest. Your internal circuits need exercise to run efficiently and if you deprive your physical and mental, of this, it will interfere with settling down for a long winter's nap.

Consequences of Sitting on the Couch with the Sweet and Salty Snacks

There's no scooting around this one. If you choose to snooze, you'll lose when it comes to exercising. The consequences are as follows…

WEIGHT GAIN – Lack of exercise greatly increases the chances of weight gain, which of course means you are on the radar for a medley of serious health issues.

SHORTENED LIFE SPAN – It goes without saying that a weaker body isn't going to live as long as a strong one. Exercise on a routine basis makes the body strong.

INCREASED SUCCESPTIBLITY TO ILLNESS AND DISEASE – Exercising releases all sorts of positive chemicals into the body that help keep diseases and minor aches and pains at bay. Less creaks and cracks and most definitely less serious disease, like heart disease, stroke and diabetes.

MENTAL CLOUDINESS – You snooze you lose here. Lack of exercise is also going to affect your mental positioning. You'll be less optimistic about life in general, with thoughts and basic thinking a whole lot cloudier.
If this isn't enough of an incentive to get your body moving I'm throwing my hands up! You are important and if you care about you, then you better get that butt of yours moving EVERY DAY!

So How Much Exercise Does Your Mind and Body Need?

Of course, there's a whole whack of variety here. Some bodies are programmed to utilize the benefits of exercising better than others. How much you focus, how hard you work and your specific exercises of choice all factor into specifically how much exercise your body needs at this specific moment in time. Its diverse and ever-changing.

BUT...
According to the PGFA (Physical Guidelines for Americans) it's recommended you give your body a minimum of 2.5 hours of moderate to intense cardiovascular activity each week. This doesn't mean strolling around the block or coasting on your Mary Poppins pretty, pink, bike with flowers and a basket. It means exercising like you mean it, pushing yourself and working up a sweat. Does your body good, not to mention your noggin!

When you think about it, that's just 30 minutes 5 days a week. Ideally you'll want to work this up to closer to an hour 5-6 days a week.

What's as or maybe more important in weight training or strength training exercises. This should happen 2-3 days a week for at least 15 minutes each session. Building muscle helps blast fat, strengthen your body, increase metabolism and help your body run more efficiently. Diversity is key, not only in the exercises you choose, but in level of intensity, duration, tempo, technique and rhythm. When keeping your mind and body guessing you are going to maximize your results regardless of the exercise. Don't ever forget that!

My Thoughts...
I don't want to slip into the lecture zone. Your body is made to exercise. It wants you to exercise it and if you don't, health troubles will eventually come around and take you down. Start slow and figure out what you enjoy. Play with that because honestly, exercise isn't supposed to be like getting tossed in the torture chamber. Take it from me. It really can be a whole lot of fun!

The 30 Day Shred Diet

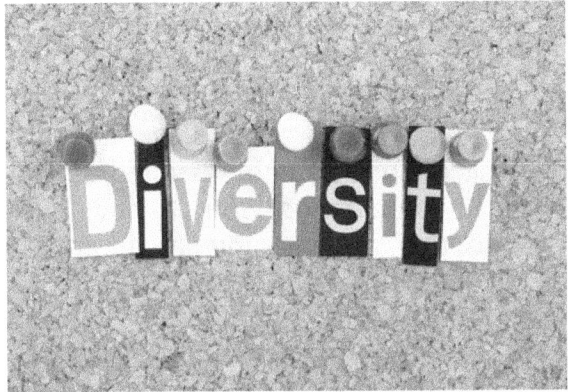

This 30 day exercise regimen concept is all over the air-waves by Jillian Michael's. In basics it focuses on a diversity scheme that confuses the body to encourage more effective calorie and fat burn. 3-2-1 is the system, the ration of weight training, and cardiovascular exercise to abdominal work. For example, 3 minutes of pull-ups and pushups, 2 minutes hard running, and 1 minute of alternating crunches and oblique's.

Makes sense here because strength training and muscle building have moved front and center stage when it comes to blasting fat and keeping it off. This diverse circuit is completed 3 times with a proper warm up and cool down. Very important because the last thing you want is serious injury.

There are 3 stages of this Shred Diet. Each is done for 10 days.

STAGE ONE – Lots of pushups, squats, lunges and weighted arm exercises for the strength training. Shadow boxing, jumping jacks and butt kicks are examples of the cardio. Crunches, lower abs and oblique's are the abdominal portion.

Note: If you haven't exercised at all you WILL feel this. It WILL hurt, but keep in mind it gets better!

STAGE TWO – Now you're set to push your body some. The intensity picks up. Strength training gets more challenging, along with abdominal work. It may not seem quite so hard though, because the first 10 days helped you "condition" your body to work hard.

STAGE THREE – Again, everything increases in intensity. With the cardio portion of this stage you also incorporate more strength training. A challenge, but by this point you're certainly ready for it. Weights are used when shadow boxing, butt kicking and executing jumping jacks.

The idea of the program is to shock your system, keep the exercises diversified and maximize your body in the fat burning process. It's a great start buy unless you look to eating healthy too. You aren't going to lose any weight. That's a fact!

Pluses???
Cheap-Cheap-Cheap!
You really don't have to pay a penny if you're innovative here. No equipment is absolutely essential and you can actually find the program on-line if you're willing to search. So it's all there if you know what you're searching for! That's gotta be a big plus!

You'll Feel It

I guess you could view this as a good or bad thing. But by feeling sore you "know" things are changing. A signal your body is working hard to get into shape and the aches and pains you are feeling is just the rust working out of your system. "Feeling" it happening is good as gold in the incentive department.

Stay Put To Get Comfortable
Again, it's a double edge sword here. But being able to get the kinks out in the comfort of your own home is often just what people need to build up the confidence in their look to step outside the house and get into some serious training, one step at a time and if the first few steps need to happen in-house, then that's what you have to do!

Short and Sweet – No Excuses
Anybody can find 20-30 minutes in the day to exercise. You just make the choice and do it. There's no huge 2 hour commitment that might scare off those sitting nervously on the fence. This time-frame is peanuts and definitely doable!

Believable Time Frame
For some people, taking a 3 month exercise session or committing to something long-term right off the hop is difficult, a deterrent because their vision of being healthy and in shape just isn't believable yet. This very small level of commitment makes the first step easier. Get yourself used to this and you'll be more open to future changes, which is all a part of the program of getting healthy for life. An open mind to changing and constantly challenging yourself just "is."

Set To Your Level
Each session can easily be modified to your current fitness level. So there are no excuses that it's "too hard," or "you just can't keep up!" The idea is to be true to you and

always make sure you are challenging you. That part of the equation is completely in your hands because going through the motions is just cheating yourself.

With a flip there's always a flop...

Minuses???

Social Neglect

Honestly, it's really not healthy to stay in and exercise. By getting out there and getting social as you are powering your way into shape. You are solidifying your health commitment to you and have others around you that will hold you to it. It's so easy to let yourself down. To just roll over, switch off the alarm and fall back into your deep and dreamy sleep, instead of getting your butt out of bed to get that heart pumping. Exercising at home has this huge hurdle to jump.

Technique Issues

Unfortunately, technique when exercising can make or break your workout. Particularly if you are just beginning, proper technique is essential for optimal results. Having a trainer or exercise instructor right beside you to watch and ensure you are keeping your back straight and butt out on squats, that's you're not dropping your belly to the floor and arching your back on pushups, is so very important.

It's not that you can't well with the 30 Day Shred Diet. You just have to pay careful attention to how you are executing ALL the time. Hope this makes sense?

A great tip here is to watch yourself if you can in the mirror practicing. Paying attention to the exercises and focusing on the muscles being used. It can only help!

Repetition May Allow the Mind to Wander

It's not that you're going to get bored with this exercise regimen. But it is very repetitive. For some, initially they really like this. Others, it's not such a good thing. You may find a weird sense of comfort in it or you may use it to daydream a little.

MAIN ISSUE OF CONCERN WITH 30 DAY SHRED DIET?

If you're looking to build lean muscle, tone and strengthen and lose weight. Then you are going to have to eat healthier. Your eating habits are going to have to match your deep desire to get fit. If you're seriously committed for life to lose that last 10-20 pounds, you're going to have to eat well for life. And it's not about restrictive dieting. That frame of mind will set you up to fail. It's about making better food choices in life that in time will turn into a habit.

Solution?

Incorporate healthy eating strategies while you're exercising with the 30 Day Shred Diet. This communicates to your body you are serious about blasting fat, getting fit and making healthier food choices for life! It's a choice and it's yours to make.

Don't worry. You're not going to be left hanging here. About the eating…

My Thoughts…
As you can see we just scooted over the concept of the 30 Day Shred Diet here. The idea being this is an introductory book and I'd rather get the basics straight here instead of complicating things by getting too detailed and frilly on you. There are good's and bad's with this exercise regimen. It's important you take what works for you and add it to your master plan. Or perhaps, start with this program and decide after completing at least one round of it how you like it. Nothing is written in stone and you can modify anything you like at any time with the focus of

getting your body and mind in tip-top shape while shed-ding fat faster! You CAN do it!

The Shred Diet – The Eating End of the Equation

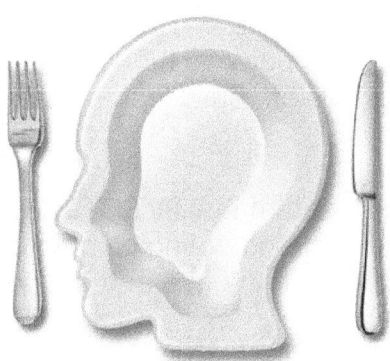

FACT: If you want to lose weight, get toned and rock hard sexy and stay that way for life. You're going to have to eat healthy! You can accept and embrace that one or just continue on as you are.

As mentioned previously, Dr. Ian K. Smith is known for the concept of "The Shred Diet," with the idea of continuously tricking the body and mind to ensure constant calorie burning, enabling you to break that body plateau and blast through that last bothersome 10-20 pounds of fat.

Often, people get stuck in what I call a weight-loss rut. I'm sure you've been here before. Where you're seemingly doing all the "right" things and just can't drop anymore weight if your body gets used to your boring workout routine such as the same length, tempo, intensity, weights and cardio exercise. And your diet is one in the same day after day, year after year. Chances are crazy high that you're going to hit a brick wall and stop seeing results. At this point many people throw in the towel YOU are not going to!

This Shred Diet teaches healthy, smart eating that's diverse in nature on purpose. Focusing on low sugar eating, meal replacements and set meal spacing. This keeps confusing your body so that it keeps working with you to burn your rolls off, build lean muscle and get you skinny!

This is a 6 week program that includes detox, cleansing and various strategic food eating combinations to help kick your metabolism in the butt and get your body lean and svelte.

The claim is you'll lose about twenty pounds or 4 inches in this 6 week program.
This Shred Diet eating strategy goes in cycles of 6 weeks. Once you've finished a cycle if you still need to drop more fat you just start another cycle. These cycle weeks are each labelled and you get to choose which to use after completing your first full cycle.
Here are a few basics with this diet just to give you an idea of the layout.

First Week – Prime – Here you are learning about why meal spacing is important, tips to smart snacking and helping to teach you hunger to get satiated without pigging out. One liquid meal – protein shake, smoothie or soup. Eat fruit or veggie with. Low-calories meals with meal plan. Low-calorie snacks. I alcohol drink twice a week limit. Carbs – 2 slices whole grain bread during day.

Second Week – Challenge – Moving into the groove, it's now important to challenge yourself. Here you will get rid of bad eating habits and open your mind to creating new healthy eating habits to replace them. Make the decision and do it for life. Two smoothies, protein shakes or soup per day, low-calorie. Eat each with fruit or veggies. Other meals strict in calories as per meal plan. Low-calorie snacks under 100 calories. Alcohol 1 drink per week.

Third Week – Transformation – This is the hardest of the Shred Diet. You'll have three low-calorie liquid meals per day with the fruit of veggies. Low-calorie snacks. Limited alcohol and lemon water.

Fourth Week – Ascend - Two low-calorie smoothies, protein shakes or soup. Eat with fruit or vegetables. With the meals you follow the fairly strict guidelines, but get to choose a few higher calories. As always diversity is key. Snacks low-calorie. Alcohol limited and lemon water with breakfast to get your metabolism kicking.

Fifth Week – Cleanse – Low-calorie smoothie, protein shake or soup per day with veggies or fruit. Eat meals according to meal plan. A few more variations here are allotted for snacks. One cup lemon water with breakfast. One cup cranberry juice and hibiscus tea each day. No alcohol.

Sixth Week – Explode – One shake, smoothie or soup per day, low-calorie. With fruit or veggies. Follow the strict meal plan. Snacks vary in diversity and calories. Alcohol limit to 3 glasses of wine per week, or 3 glasses of beer or mixed drink twice a week. Three slices whole grain bread per day anytime.

Benefits
-Lowers risk for light blood pressure and diabetes

-Aids in weight loss and control
-Increases energy levels
-Improved overall life outlook

Pluses
-Numerous meals per day, up to seven
-Real food eaten
-Not expensive and food combinations increase energy
-Great if looking to lose ten or fifty pounds

Minuses
-If you stop and change your ways the fat can pack right back on
-Tedious to get all meals in your tummy if you work with a tight schedule
-Generally works with your preferences and tolerances or it doesn't, hit or miss
BASIC ISSUES?

Having this diet run in 6 week cycles plants "temporary" in the brain instead of forever. If you are going to lose weight and keep it off the mindset has to be diet changes for life, not 6 weeks.

Without focuses on regular fitness activity this diet isn't worth the space it takes up in your brain. The Shred Diet concept as a whole basically makes sense, but it needs to be incorporated into a healthy lifestyle if the weight loss portion is going to stick. As it stands it just sets you up for another fad diet, misleading to those new to learning effective weight loss.

My Thoughts…
I may have dove into this eating strategy a little deeper than initially intended. But you can see there is a little bit of complexity to it. The basic idea behind the Shred Diet makes sense. But that really doesn't matter if you can't

commit to learning this eating plan, sticking with it and opening your mind to making changes where you see fit. Take from this eating program what works for you, your body, preferences and tolerances and you're cruising along just fine.

Action Steps

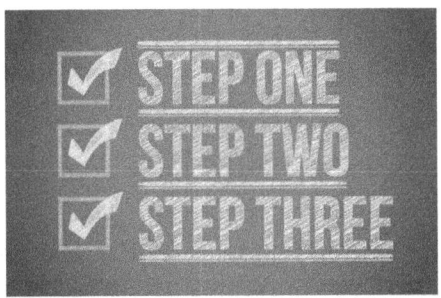

One-Create Plan
Without a solid long-term weight loss plan written down on paper, you're just out of luck in the middle of the ocean, in a flimsy Strawberry Shortcake rubber dingy with a hole, no paddle, a cut on your leg and hungry Great Whites nearby!

You need a plan of action that details both the eating and exercise goals you've made. Using the 30 Day Shred Diet to cover the initial exercise portion of your plan is a smart move. Adding to that, the Shred Diet eating strategy, you are definitely headed toward "Lean-ville."

Here you need to keep your mind open and make sure you gear your plan of action toward your tolerance and preferences. Set yourself up for success and get help from a professional or at least run your plan past them to ensure you've got everything covered.

This is going to take some time because this diet and exercise regimen has a lot of diversity. Meaning you'll have to give yourself time to get used to the layout of your plan. Don't allow frustration to get the best of you. Stick with your plan and you WILL get results that make you smile.

Two-Set Yourself Up For Success
It's too easy just to go through the motions, not put in all you've got, and set yourself up to fail. It's an excuse to throw in the towel and revert back to lazy and unhealthy ways of days past. If that's what you want to do, that's your choice.

For those of you that truly want to make your new flab loss stick, you need to just decide it's going to happen and it will. Be true to yourself here and ensure you are gearing your exercise routine to what you do and don't like. For instance, if you can't seem to ever wake up before noon, don't try and schedule your exercise for 6am each day. That's just a disaster waiting to happen. Make it for after lunch or maybe when works done. This increases your shot at sticking with it and that means you're more likely to make healthy life choices with your exercise that stick for life.

The same does with eating. You can always make substitutions. It just may take a little digger to find out what works. Take the time to do this if there are foods that just don't work with your system or taste buds. Even when you're watching what you're eating, you've gotta enjoy it! Having supports in place also help here. Tell your friends and family about what you're doing. If you need to get a health professional involved to ensure you stay on track, do it! Want to lose that last 20 pounds with a partner, all the better. The idea is if others have expectations, you're going to reach your goals. Chances are better that you will!

Having regular check-ins with your progress is also important. Whether it's a journal or just once a month where

44

you step on the scale. The important point here is that you are seeing results and recording them. Seeing is believing and this will intrinsically motivate you to want more!

Three-Implement and Maintain – Tips to Succeed
You need to actually take action if you want to get results. Many people get over prepared. Trying to get everything set up perfectly and when it comes time to actually implement, they just don't bother. Doesn't make sense, but it's easy to do. You're better off to jump right in and get going, adjusting to better your eating and exercise decisions as you move along.

Now I can give you oodles of tips for maintaining your weight loss once you've hit your targets. To simplify, it you need to keep doing what you are doing and make these healthy changes for life. It's not about dieting and exercising on and off for the rest of your life. Not unless you just want to keep yo-yoing with your fat loss.

Stick with what works for you! Sensible eating and exercising for life is your goal. To ensure you stay on track, have a set weight you don't want to go above no matter what. So let's say you got your weight down to 130 pounds. Your max weight might be 135lbs. If you creep back up to that weight that's your signal to bear down, tighten up on your eating and exercising until you drop back down a few pounds. You can keep this in check by stepping on the scale once a week just to be sure. Does that make sense?

The last thing you want to do is let yourself creep back out of control again and all your hard effort is wasted. It's up to you to ensure that doesn't happen. You CAN do it!

Tips for Success in Weight Loss

COMMIT

Both you and I know that if you want to reach your weight loss goal and keep it permanent you are going to have to create healthy eating and exercise habits for life. This is a permanent thing and requires the same mindset. Life is going to whack you with stresses and all sorts of pressures that will test your newfound ways. Expect this and stand strong against them. If you choose to seriously commit and succeed, you will.

BE REALISTIC

The more real you are in your goals and expectations, the more success you will enjoy, for instance, if you're headed away on a holiday with a bunch of your girlfriends, don't expect to keep dropping pounds like you have been staying tight with your regimen at home. You know that isn't likely to happen. So, why not just try hard to maintain what you've lost for that week and get back on track when you're home? That's a realistic expectation that will prevent you from throwing in the towel. Understand when you initially start your weight loss programs you're shocking your system and likely going to drop quite a few pounds right off that bat. Don't expect this pace to continue because it will slow and find its own rhythm. You've just got to stick with it and go with the ups and downs. That's being smart and realistic.

GET MOTIVATED

Unless you REALLY want to lose weight and keep it off for good. The chances are pretty great that you're going to end getting unmotivated and back into your fat chair. Change is hard and it's important you get motivated from the inside out. Perhaps, you want to slip into your teeny weeny yellow polka-dot bikini by summer time? Or maybe you've got a fabulous sexy hot slinky black dress that's always been too small, that you would love to get your body back into in time for your sister's wedding?

Just make sure you've got strong reasons and motivations to get that fat off for good. The stronger, the better here.

My Thoughts…
It really doesn't matter if you're the smartest exercise and nutrition expert on the planet. If you aren't going to take the information in your noggin and apply it to your everyday life, it's useless! Don't wait. The best time for you to get started is right now. Take a big leap and worry about the "what ifs" another day!

Exercise Myths

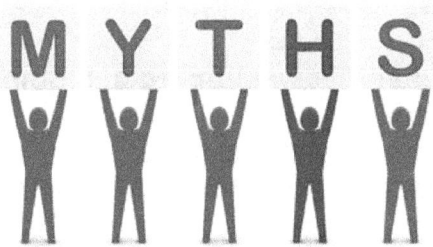

Don't freak out here on me, but you may be hugely surprised how many supposed "facts" you think you know about getting fit, really are fiction! Don't feel bad though. Particularly if you're just getting your feet wet in the exercise department. It's natural to trust what other people say to a point, particularly when they are in better shape than you.

False information in the workout room is only going to make your journey to optimum fitness harder. Here are a few exercise facts in disguise. They really are fiction.

Myth One: Getting your cardiovascular in on the treadmill is much better for your body than jogging on pavement.
Truth: It doesn't matter how you slice it here. Running is a hard impact workout, taking its toll over time on your knees, hips and joints. There isn't much difference what

hard surface you are running on, although, a soft sandy surface is better than a hard pavement.

You're best to switch it up here so you aren't always running to get your heart rate pumping. Maybe run twice a week and bike, swim, or use the Stairmaster the other days. You want you to be careful with your body. Work it hard, but beware of overdoing it. Wear and tear is wear and tear, right?

Myth Two: You'll get washboard abs doing a hundred crunches a day!
Truth: In your dreams! Sure the crunches are going to help strengthen your abdominal muscles. But that's not going to get you a six-pack! First off you have six main abdominal muscles and you need to exercise them all separately to get that ripped look. Next up, it's important to understand unless you have an ultra low body fat percentage. It doesn't matter how much ab work you do. You aren't going to see any rippling till you get that extra body fat off you and step into you fittest of the fit lean suit! We are talking at least below 10%.

Myth Three: You better have a sports drink during exercise to replace those lost electrolytes.
Truth: Oh, what a tangled marketing web we weave. Blame this one on all those sports drinks you see famous sports figures gulping back when captured on camera. For the average person, exercise 1-2 hours a day, the only thing your body needs is water in the hydration department. Why? Well, because you aren't working your body long enough or hard enough to zap all your readily available energy supplies. Save the power drinks and bars for the athletes that exercise at incredibly high intensity levels for hours on end. Drink water and never mind the other stuff!

Myth Four: Stretch before you exercise and you won't ever get injured.
Truth: Whoa...just a minute here. This is one of those comments that gives you a false sense of security. Sure, it's important to warm your muscles up before you exercise. But if you start stretching too aggressively when your muscles are cold, you WILL injure yourself. Experts agree it's best to warm up first doing a light jog or hopping on the bike for 5 minutes at a moderate pace BEFORE you begin gently stretching. This way your muscles are warm and stretch easier. Think of it like warming up an elastic band before stretching it. You don't want it to break now do you?

Myth Five: If you work out you're just going to build muscle and not lose fat.
Truth: This one is all dependent on how much you are exercising and what you're eating. If you're looking to lose weight and consume fewer calories while exercising. Then you're not likely to gain weight even though you're building muscle with your weight training. The idea that lean muscle burns more fat and calories than fat does is appealing to people that want to get toned and lose weight. Sure muscle weighs more than fat, but the difference is minimal, if you are executing a balanced health plan. Including cardiovascular activity, weight training and healthy eating choices, you should have no trouble building sexy lean muscle, building strength and zapping those cottage cheese thighs.

Myth Six: Exercising when older is just dangerous.
Truth: This one is just FALSE! There isn't one single health professional out there that will advise you not to exercise because of your age. It doesn't matter your health condition, previous exercise experience or your age. ANY kind of exercise is going to be good for your body and mind. Sure, if you have knee problems you

51

might need to modify your squats or do half lunges instead. If you have had a hip replacement you're not going to get your cardio on the treadmill. But you can get it swimming or on the bike. Where there's a will there's a way. And the advantages of regular exercise are so freaking high they run over any sort of excuse you can think of.

My Thoughts…
Starting a new exercise regimen with the cold hard facts is only going to kick you in the right direction. If something doesn't make sense to you when exercising, make sure you take the time to find out if it's fact or foe. It'll likely save you a whole lot of time and nasty frustrations on your path to getting that sexy body you've been hiding for so long.

Nutrition Myths

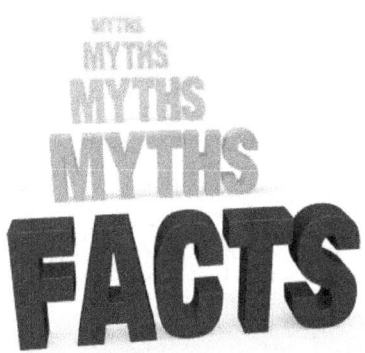

As with the exercise side of the coin, nutrition myths are running rampant in our world today. And it doesn't take much to convince yourself to believe a myth really is the truth, particularly if it makes your path to healthy eating easier. Time to shed some light on these vampires and watch them burn!

Myth One: Having a chicken burger instead of the real deal is wise of you.
Truth: Sure, there are very healthy chicken burgers. But that's only if the bread is whole grain. The chicken is grilled and not pumped full of hormones and who knows what else. And that you don't load your burger with fattening toppings like cheese, mayo and other creamy dressings.

Unfortunately, in most cases, it's actually healthier to have a plain burger than the chicken variety. Having just TWO tablespoons of mayo no your chicken burger adds 200 calories of pure fat. Never mind the chicken and bun!

Be careful with your pre-programed thinking that chicken is better for you than beef. Often, that's just not the case.

Myth Two: Brown eggs are healthier than white.
Truth: Not sure what yahoo came up with this one, but it's so false! The color of the egg shell has nothing to do with the nutrient value of the egg. The eggs are different colors because of the type of hen that lays them! You are best to choose organic and "free range" when gathering your eggs. This just means they are void of harmful pesticides and hormones often injected into chickens to optimize their growth for the purpose of being cost-effective.

Myth Three: Butter makes you fat.
Truth: No one food or group of food makes you fat. It's the combination of how much you eat and how many calories your body burns regularly. Any food can make you fat if you eat too much. Avocados are healthy, right? Well, if you sat on your butt all day and ate 25 avocados, I can pretty much guarantee you're going to get a little tubby.
Be smart about the quantity of food you eat and you won't have to worry so much about padding your extra tires.

Myth Four: Eating meat is going to make you fat.
Truth: Not true! Your body needs protein to build lean muscle and help maintain the health of your cells. Protein helps your brain function and your skin, nails and hair beautiful. 2-3 servings of lean protein are suggested every day, a little more if you are focusing on weight training. The old school of thought was to stay away from meat and get skinny. The new school of thought is to eat lean meat in moderation to rev up your metabolism, build lean muscle, blast fat and get energized. Need I say more?

Myth Five: Carbs will make you tubby.
Truth: Your body uses carbohydrates for long term energy. Eating complex carbs in moderation gives your body the essential vitamins and minerals it requires, along with fiber to help keep you regular, pushing toxic substances out of your system so it can run cleaner.

Where people muck up is choosing simple sugar carbs like white bread, pasta, pastries, cookies and other sweet treats. Instead, choose healthy whole grains, vegetables, beans, lentils, whole wheat pasta and brown rice. These in moderation are exactly what your body needs.

My Thoughts…
If I had a penny for every food myth I've heard, I'd be retired! Again, it's important to trust your gut when it comes to eating. If you aren't sure about something, take the time to find out the facts. The last thing you want to do is sabotage your weight loss plans because of a misstep in the nutrition department. Wouldn't you agree?

Final Thoughts

I understand this is a whole lot of information to process, absorb, sort through and take action with. What's important here is you understand there is no one diet or exercise regimen that's going to get you fit, slim, healthy and energized for life. As your days are ever-changing, so should be your eating and exercise regimen. The basic concept for the 30 Day Shred Diet exercise regimen makes sense, diversifying your workouts regularly to encourage optimal results for your efforts. The ratio of muscle building, cardio and abs makes sense. And ultimately it's up to you as to how much weight you're going to lose and how quickly. If you work harder and pay attention to all the delicious, healthy food you fill your belly with WHILE you're concentrating on regular exercise.

Then, inevitably you're going to open the lines of communication that you want to build lean muscle and blast pesky fat. Your body will oblige and do just that. My personal concern here is that this 30 Day Shred Diet exercise regimen is too secluded and short-lived. Just 30 days isn't enough time to turn anything into habit and it's incredibly tough to get motivated to work hard in your living room. But it is a start.

On the flip side of the coin, I haven't been shy about my concern for nutrition in this whole process. The 30 Day Shred Diet exercise program doesn't focus on how you should be fueling your body specifically. It's misinformation because you can be exercising 2-3 hours a day. But if you are eating fast food or consuming a few thousand calories more than your body expends in a day, you aren't going to get rid of that last bothersome pain in the butt 20-30 pounds.

I have the flip concern with the Shred Diet nutrition plan. Without regular exercise that's EFFECTIVE. It really is tough to maintain any sort of weight loss.

Both exercising and eating healthy need to become a plan for life. One that is always changing and geared specifically toward your tolerances and preferences. This means you just need to figure it out for the most part through trial and error. Enabling you to figure out what works for you and incorporating that as your new "normal." Keeping in the back of your brain that diversity is your best friend. By changing things up you'll keep both your mind and body guessing 24/7 and that means you are going to get the results you want continuously. Steering clear of frustrating plateaus and psychosomatic setbacks that are all a part of pushing ourselves to break old habits and create new healthier ones!

My advice is to get started with the 30 Day Shred Diet. Keep an open mind and use this as the first building block to your master plan, one that only you can create and make it a success for life!

In order for my books to rank and sell on Amazon they need positive reviews. If you enjoyed my book and have a few minutes to write a 3-5 line review about my book, that would really help me. Thank you :)

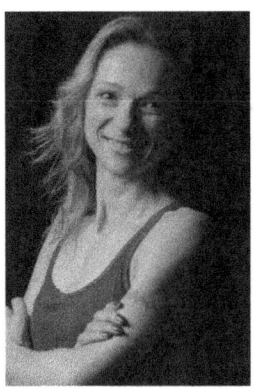

I hope that you enjoyed my book and you can check out all my other books by visiting my website at: flawlesscreativewriting.com

Disclaimer

www.ingramcontent.com/pod-product-compliance
Lightning Source LLC
Chambersburg PA
CBHW070328290526
45791CB00003B/1291